Copyright © 2018 by Dr. Thomas Richardson

All rights reserved. No part of this publication may be reproduced, distributed, or transmitted in any form or by any means, including photocopying, recording, or other electronic or mechanical methods, without the prior written permission of the publisher, except in the case of brief ☐uotations embodied in critical reviews and certain other noncommercial uses permitted by copyright law

Introduction

Lung cancer, also known as lung carcinoma is a malignant lung tumor characterized by uncontrolled cell growth in tissues of the lung. This growth can spread beyond the lung by the process of metastasis into nearby tissue or other parts of the body. Most cancers that start in the lung, known as primary lung cancers, are carcinomas. The two main types are small-cell lung carcinoma (SCLC) and non-small-cell lung carcinoma (NSCLC). The most common symptoms are coughing including coughing up blood, weight loss, shortness of breath, and chest pains.

The vast majority 85% of cases of lung cancer are due to long-term tobacco smoking. About 10–15% of cases occur in people who have never smoked.

Lung cancer was uncommon before the advent of cigarette smoking; it was not even recognized as a distinct disease until 1761. Different aspects of lung cancer were described further in 1810. Malignant lung tumors made up only 1% of all cancers seen at autopsy in 1878, but had risen to 10–15% by the early 1900s. Case reports in the medical literature numbered only 374 worldwide in 1912, but a review of autopsies showed the incidence of lung cancer had increased from 0.3% in 1852 to 5.66% in 1952 recommended smokers should stop smoking.

The connection with radon gas was first recognized among miners in the Ore Mountains near Schneeberg, Saxony. Silver has been mined there since 1470, and these mines are rich in uranium, with its accompanying radium and radon gas. Miners developed a disproportionate amount of lung disease, eventually recognized as lung cancer in the 1870s. Despite this discovery, mining continued into the 1950s, due to the USSR's demand for uranium. Radon was confirmed as a cause of lung cancer in the 1960s.

Contents

Lung cancer facts

Lung cancer is the number one cause of cancer deaths in both men and women in the U.S. and worldwide.

Cigarette smoking is the principal risk factor for development of lung cancer.

Passive exposure to tobacco smoke (passive smoking) also can cause lung cancer.

The two types of lung cancer, which grow and spread differently, are small cell lung cancers (SCLC) and non-small cell lung cancers (NSCLC).

The stage of lung cancer refers to the extent to which the cancer has spread in the body.

Treatment of lung cancer can involve a combination of surgery, chemotherapy, targeted therapy, immunotherapy, and radiation therapy as well as newer experimental methods.

The general prognosis of lung cancer is poor because doctors tend not to find the disease until it is at an advanced stage. Five-year survival is around 54% for early stage lung cancer that is localized to the lungs, but only around 4% in advanced, inoperable lung cancer.

Smoking cessation is the most important measure that can prevent the development of lung cancer.

Treatment of Stage IV Lung Cancer with ALK Rearrangement

Medications

Identification of an ALK gene rearrangement in a lung cancer is important for deciding the optimal treatment course. The ALK rearrangement means that drugs that specifically act against the abnormal fusion protein can be used. Three drugs, crizotinib (Xalkori), ceritinib (Zykadia), and alectinib (Alecensa), have been developed to target the activity of the abnormal fusion protein, and additional agents are under development. For patients with advanced or metastatic ALK-positive NSCLC who do not have metastases to the brain, the ALK inhibitor crizotinib is the recommended therapy. Ceritinib or alectinib is typically given if the cancer becomes resistant to crizotinib or if the patient is unable to tolerate crizotinib.

What is lung cancer?

Cancer of the lung, like all cancers, results from an abnormality in the body's basic unit of life, the cell. Normally, the body maintains a system of checks and balances on cell growth so that cells divide to produce new cells only when new cells are needed. Disruption of this system of checks and balances on cell growth results in an uncontrolled division and proliferation of cells that eventually forms a mass known as a tumor.

Tumors can be benign or malignant; when we speak of "cancer," we are referring to those tumors that are malignant. Benign tumors usually can be removed and do not spread to other parts of the body. Malignant tumors, on the other hand, often grow aggressively locally where they start, but tumor cells also can enter into the bloodstream or lymphatic system and then spread to other sites in the body. This process of spread is termed metastasis; the areas of tumor growth at these distant sites are called metastases. Since lung cancer tends to spread or metastasize very early after it forms, it is a very life-threatening cancer and one of the most difficult cancers to treat. While lung cancer can spread to any organ in the body, certain locations --

particularly the adrenal glands, liver, brain, and bones -- are the most common sites for lung cancer metastasis.

 The lung also is a very common site for metastasis from malignant tumors in other parts of the body. Tumor metastases are made up of the same types of cells as the original (primary) tumor. For example, if prostate cancer spreads via the bloodstream to the lungs, it is metastatic prostate cancer in the lung and is not lung cancer.

The principal function of the lungs is to exchange gases between the air we breathe and the blood. Through the lung, carbon dioxide is removed from the bloodstream and oxygen enters the bloodstream. The right lung has three lobes, while the left lung is divided into two lobes and a small structure called the lingula that is the equivalent of the middle lobe on the right. The major airways entering the lungs are the bronchi, which arise from the trachea, which is outside the lungs. The bronchi branch into progressively smaller airways called bronchioles that end in tiny sacs known as alveoli where gas exchange occurs. The lungs and chest wall are covered with a thin layer of tissue called the pleura.

Lung cancers can arise in any part of the lung, but 90%-95% of cancers of the lung are thought to arise from the epithelial cells, the cells lining the larger and smaller airways (bronchi and bronchioles); for this reason, lung cancers are sometimes called bronchogenic cancers or bronchogenic carcinomas. (Carcinoma is another term for cancer.) Cancers also can arise from the pleura (called mesotheliomas) or rarely from supporting tissues within the lungs, for example, the blood vessels.

How common is lung cancer?

Lung cancer is the most common cause of death due to cancer in both men and women throughout the world. Statistics from the American Cancer Society estimated that in 2018 there will be about 244,000 new cases of lung cancer in the U.S. occurred and over 154,000 deaths were due to the disease. According to the U.S. National Cancer Institute, approximately 6.5% of men and women in the U.S. will be diagnosed with cancer of the lung at some point in their lifetime based on data from 2011-13.

Lung cancer is predominantly a disease of the elderly; almost 70% of people diagnosed with lung cancer are over 65 years of age, while less than 3% of lung cancers occur in people under 45 years of age. The median age at diagnosis is 70 years.

Lung cancer was not common prior to the 1930s but increased dramatically over the following decades as tobacco smoking increased. In many developing countries, the incidence of lung cancer is beginning to fall following public education about the dangers of cigarette smoking and the introduction of effective smoking-cessation programs. Nevertheless, lung cancer remains among the most common types of cancers in both men and women worldwide. In the U.S., lung cancer has surpassed breast cancer as the most common cause of cancer-related deaths in women.

What are the causes and risk factors for lung cancer?

Smoking

The incidence of lung cancer is strongly correlated with cigarette smoking, with about 90% of lung cancers arising as a result of tobacco use. The risk of lung cancer increases with the number of cigarettes smoked and the time over which smoking has occurred; doctors refer to this risk in terms of pack-years of smoking history (the number of packs of cigarettes smoked per day multiplied by the number of years smoked). For example, a person who has smoked two packs of cigarettes per day for 10 years has a 20 pack-year smoking history. While the risk of lung cancer is increased with even a 10-pack-year smoking history, those with 30-pack-year histories or more are considered to have the greatest risk for the development of lung cancer. Among those who smoke two or more packs of cigarettes per day, one in seven will die of lung cancer.

Pipe and cigar smoking also can cause lung cancer, although the risk is not as high as with cigarette smoking. Thus, while someone who smokes one pack of cigarettes per day has a risk for the development of lung cancer that is 25 times higher than a nonsmoker, pipe and cigar smokers have a risk of lung cancer that is about five times that of a nonsmoker.

Tobacco smoke contains over 4,000 chemical compounds, many of which have been shown to be cancer-causing or carcinogenic. The two primary carcinogens in tobacco smoke are chemicals known as nitrosamines and polycyclic aromatic hydrocarbons. The risk of developing lung cancer decreases each year following smoking cessation as normal cells grow and replace damaged cells in the lung. In former smokers, the risk of developing lung cancer begins to approach that of a nonsmoker about 15 years after cessation of smoking.

Passive smoking

Passive smoking or the inhalation of tobacco smoke by nonsmokers who share living or working quarters with smokers, also is an established risk factor for the development of lung cancer. Research has shown that nonsmokers who reside with a smoker have a 24% increase in risk for developing lung cancer when compared with nonsmokers who do not reside with a smoker. The risk appears to increase with the degree of exposure (number of years exposed and number of cigarettes smoked by the household partner) to secondhand smoke.

Exposure to asbestos fibers
Asbestos fibers are silicate fibers that can persist for a lifetime in lung tissue following exposure to asbestos. The workplace was a common source of exposure to asbestos fibers, as asbestos was widely used in the past as both thermal and acoustic insulation. Today, asbestos use is limited or banned in many countries, including the U.S. Both lung cancer and mesothelioma (cancer of the pleura of the lung as well as of the lining of the abdominal cavity called the peritoneum) are associated with exposure to asbestos. Cigarette smoking drastically increases the chance of developing an asbestos-related lung cancer in workers exposed to asbestos; asbestos workers who do not smoke have a fivefold greater risk of developing lung cancer than nonsmokers, but asbestos workers who smoke have a risk that is fifty- to ninety-fold greater than nonsmokers.

Exposure to radon gas

Radon gas is a natural radioactive gas that is a natural decay product of uranium that emits a type of ionizing radiation. Radon gas is a known cause of lung cancer, with an estimated 12% of lung cancer deaths attributable to radon gas, or about 21,000 lung-cancer-related deaths annually in the U.S., making radon the second leading cause of lung cancer in the U.S. after smoking. As with asbestos exposure, concomitant smoking greatly increases the risk of lung cancer with radon exposure. Radon gas can travel up through soil and enter homes through gaps in the foundation, pipes, drains, or other openings.

Other causes lung cancer?

Familial predisposition
While the majority of lung cancers are associated with tobacco smoking, the fact that not all smokers eventually develop lung cancer suggests that other factors, such as individual genetic susceptibility, may play a role in the causation of lung cancer. Numerous studies have shown that lung cancer is more likely to occur in both smoking and nonsmoking relatives of those who have had lung cancer

than in the general population. It is unclear how much of this risk is due to shared environmental factors (like a smoking household) and how much is related to genetic risk. People who inherit certain genes, like genes that interfere with DNA repair, may be at greater risk for several types of cancer. Tests to identify people at increased genetic risk of lung cancer are not yet available for routine use.

Lung diseases

The presence of certain diseases of the lung, notably chronic obstructive pulmonary disease (COPD), is associated with an increased risk (four- to six-fold the risk of a nonsmoker) for the development of lung cancer even after the effects of concomitant cigarette smoking are excluded. Pulmonary fibrosis (scarring of the lung) appears to increase the risk about seven-fold, and this risk does not appear to be related to smoking.

Prior history of lung cancer

Survivors of lung cancer have a greater risk of developing a second lung cancer than the general population has of developing a first lung cancer. Survivors of non-small cell lung cancers (NSCLCs, see below) have an additive risk of 1%-2% per year for developing a second lung cancer. In survivors of small cell lung cancers (SCLCs, see below), the risk for development of second lung cancers approaches 6% per year.

Air pollution

Air pollution from vehicles, industry, and power plants can raise the likelihood of developing lung cancer in exposed individuals. Up to 1%-2% of lung cancer deaths are attributable to breathing polluted air, and experts believe that prolonged exposure to highly polluted air can carry a risk for the development of lung cancer similar to that of passive smoking.

Exposure to diesel exhaust

Exhaust from diesel engines is made up of gases and soot (particulate matter). Many occupations, such as truck drivers, toll booth workers, forklift and other heavy machinery operators, railroad and dock workers, miners, garage workers and mechanics, and some farm workers are fre□uently exposed to diesel exhaust. Studies of workers exposed to diesel exhaust have shown a small but significant increase in the risk of developing lung cancer.

What are the types of lung cancer?

Lung cancers, also known as bronchogenic carcinomas because they arise from the bronchi within the lungs, are broadly classified into two types: small cell lung cancers (SCLC) and non-small cell lung cancers (NSCLC). This classification is based upon the microscopic appearance of the tumor cells themselves, specifically the size of the cells. These two types of cancers grow and spread in different ways and may have different treatment options, so a distinction between these two types is important.

SCLC comprise about 20% of lung cancers and are the most aggressive and rapidly growing of all lung cancers. SCLC are strongly related to cigarette smoking, with only 1% of these tumors occurring in nonsmokers. SCLC metastasize rapidly to many sites within the body and are most often discovered after they have spread extensively. Referring to a specific cell appearance often seen when examining samples of SCLC under the microscope, these cancers are sometimes called oat cell carcinomas.

NSCLC are the most common lung cancers, accounting for about 80% of all lung cancers. NSCLC can be divided into several main types that are named based upon the type of cells found in the tumor:

Adenocarcinomas are the most commonly seen type of NSCLC in the U.S. and comprise up to 50% of NSCLC. While adenocarcinomas are associated with smoking like other lung cancers, this type is observed as well in nonsmokers who develop lung cancer. Most adenocarcinomas arise in the outer, or peripheral, areas of the lungs.

Bronchioloalveolar carcinoma is a subtype of adenocarcinoma that freuently develops at multiple sites in the lungs and spreads along the preexisting alveolar walls.

Squamous cell carcinomas were formerly more common than adenocarcinomas; at present, they account for about 30% of NSCLC. Also, known as epidermoid carcinomas, suamous cell cancers arise most fre□uently in the central chest area in the bronchi.

Large cell carcinomas, sometimes referred to as undifferentiated carcinomas, are the least common type of NSCLC.

Mixtures of different types of NSCLC also are seen.

Other types of cancers can arise in the lung; these types are much less common than NSCLC and SCLC and together comprise only 5%-10% of lung cancers:

Bronchial carcinoids account for up to 5% of lung cancers. These tumors are sometimes referred to as lung neuroendocrine tumors. They are generally small (3 cm-4 cm or less) when diagnosed and occur most commonly in people under 40 years of age. Unrelated to cigarette smoking, carcinoid tumors can metastasize, and a small proportion of these tumors secrete hormone-like substances that may cause specific symptoms related to the hormone being produced. Carcinoids generally grow and spread more slowly than bronchogenic cancers, and many are detected early enough to be amenable to surgical resection.

Cancers of supporting lung tissue such as smooth muscle, blood vessels, or cells involved in the immune response can rarely occur in the lung.

What are lung cancer symptoms and signs?

Everything You Need to Know About Lung Cancer

- Stages
- Symptoms
- Back Pain
- Causes
- Risks
- Smoking
- Diagnosis
- Treatment
- Home Remedies
- Diet
- Life Expectancy
- Facts

Are there different types of lung cancer?

Lung cancer is cancer that starts in the lungs.

The most common type is non-small cell lung cancer (NSCLC). NSCLC makes up about 80 to 85 percent of all cases. Thirty percent of these start in the cells that form the lining of the body's cavities and surfaces. This type usually forms in the outer part of the lungs (adenocarcinomas). Another 30 percent begins in cells that line the passages of the respiratory tract (squamous cell carcinoma).

A rare subset of adenocarcinoma begins in the tiny air sacs in the lungs (alveoli). It's called adenocarcinoma in situ (AIS). This type isn't aggressive and may not invade surrounding tissue or need immediate treatment. Faster-growing types of NSCLC include large-cell carcinoma and large-cell neuroendocrine tumors.

Small-cell lung cancer (SCLC) represents about 15 to 20 percent of lung cancers. SCLC grows and spreads faster than NSCLC. This also makes it more likely to respond to chemotherapy, but it's also less likely to be cured with treatment.

In some cases, lung cancer tumors contain both NSCLC and SCLC cells.

Mesothelioma is another type of lung cancer. It's usually associated with asbestos exposure. Carcinoid tumors start in hormone producing (neuroendocrine) cells.

Tumors in the lungs can grow □uite large before you notice symptoms. Early symptoms mimic a cold or other common conditions, so most people don't seek medical attention right away. That's one reason why lung cancer isn't usually diagnosed in an early stage.

Stages of lung cancer

Cancer stages tell how far the cancer has spread and help guide treatment. The chance of successful or curative treatment is much higher when lung cancer is diagnosed and treated in the early stages, before it spreads. Because lung cancer doesn't cause obvious symptoms in the earlier stages, diagnosis often comes after it has spread.

Non-small cell lung cancer has four main stages:

Stage 1: Cancer is found in the lung, but it has not spread outside the lung.

Stage 2: Cancer is found in the lung and nearby lymph nodes.

Stage 3: Cancer is in the lung and lymph nodes in the middle of the chest.

Stage 3A: Cancer is found in lymph nodes, but only on the same side of the chest where cancer first started growing.

Stage 3B: Cancer has spread to lymph nodes on the opposite side of the chest or to lymph nodes above the collarbone.

Stage 4: Cancer has spread to both lungs, into the area around the lungs, or to distant organs.

Small-cell lung cancer (SCLC) has two main stages. In the limited stage, cancer is found in only one lung or nearby lymph nodes on the same side of the chest.

The extensive stage means cancer has spread:

- throughout one lung
- to the opposite lung
- to lymph nodes on the opposite side
- to fluid around the lung
- to bone marrow
- to distant organs

At the time of diagnosis, 2 out of 3 people with SCLC are already in the extensive stage.

What are the symptoms of lung cancer?

Symptoms of non-small cell lung cancer and small cell lung cancer are basically the same.

Early symptoms may include:

- lingering or worsening cough
- coughing up phlegm or blood
- chest pain that worsens when you breathe deeply, laugh, or cough
- hoarseness
- shortness of breath
- wheezing
- weakness and fatigue
- loss of appetite and weight loss

You might also have recurrent respiratory infections such as pneumonia or bronchitis.

As cancer spreads, additional symptoms depend on where new tumors form. For example, if in the:

lymph nodes: lumps, particularly in the neck or collarbone

bones: bone pain, particularly in the back, ribs, or hips

brain or spine: headache, dizziness, balance issues, or numbness in arms or legs

liver: yellowing of skin and eyes (jaundice)

Tumors at the top of the lungs can affect facial nerves, leading to drooping of one eyelid, small pupil, or lack of perspiration on one side of the face. Together, these symptoms are called Horner syndrome. It can also cause shoulder pain.

Tumors can press on the large vein that transports blood between the head, arms, and heart. This can cause swelling of the face, neck, upper chest, and arms.

Lung cancer sometimes creates a substance similar to hormones, causing a wide variety of symptoms called paraneoplastic syndrome, which include:

- muscle weakness
- nausea
- vomiting
- fluid retention
- high blood pressure
- high blood sugar
- confusion
- seizures

- coma

Lung cancer and back pain

Back pain is fairly common in the general population. It's possible to have lung cancer and unrelated back pain. Most people with back pain don't have lung cancer.

Not everyone with lung cancer gets back pain, but many do. For some people, back pain turns out to be one of the first symptoms of lung cancer.

Back pain can be due to the pressure of large tumors growing in the lungs. It can also mean that cancer has spread to your spine or ribs. As it grows, a cancerous tumor can cause compression of the spinal cord.

 That can lead to neurologic deterioration causing:

- weakness of the arms and legs
- numbness or loss of sensation in the legs and feet
- urinary and bowel incontinence
- interference with the spinal blood supply

Without treatment, back pain caused by cancer will continue to worsen. Back pain may improve if treatment such as surgery, radiation, or chemotherapy can successfully remove or shrink the tumor.

In addition, your doctor can use corticosteroids or prescribe pain relievers such as acetaminophen and nonsteroidal anti-inflammatory drugs (NSAIDs). For more severe pain, opioids such as morphine or oxycodone may be needed.

What causes lung cancer?

Anyone can get lung cancer, but 90 percent of lung cancer cases are the result of smoking.

From the moment you inhale smoke into your lungs, it starts damaging your lung tissue. The lungs can repair the damage, but continued exposure to smoke makes it increasingly difficult for the lungs to keep up the repair. Once cells are damaged, they begin to behave abnormally, increasing the likelihood of developing lung cancer. Small-cell lung cancer is almost always associated with heavy smoking. When you stop smoking, you lower your risk of lung cancer over time.

Exposure to radon, a naturally existing radioactive gas, is the second leading cause, according to the American Lung Association.

Radon enters buildings through small cracks in the foundation. Smokers who are also exposed to radon have a very high risk of lung cancer.

Breathing in other hazardous substances, especially over a long period of time, can also cause lung cancer. A type of lung cancer called mesothelioma is almost always caused by exposure to asbestos.

Other substances that can cause lung cancer are:

- arsenic
- cadmium
- chromium
- nickel
- some petroleum products
- uranium

 Inherited genetic mutations may make you more likely to develop lung cancer, especially if you smoke or are exposed to other carcinogens.

Sometimes, there's no obvious cause for lung cancer.

Risk factors for lung cancer

The biggest risk factor for lung cancer is smoking. That includes cigarettes, cigars, and pipes. Tobacco products contain thousands of toxic substances. According to the Centers for Disease Control and Prevention (CDC), cigarette smokers are 15 to 30 times more likely to get lung cancer than nonsmokers. The longer you smoke, the greater the risk. Quitting smoking can lower that risk.

Breathing in secondhand smoke is also a major risk factor. Every year in the United States, about 7,300 people who have never smoked die from lung cancer caused by secondhand smoke.

Exposure to radon, a naturally occurring gas, increases your risk of lung cancer. Radon rises from the ground, entering buildings through small cracks. It's the leading cause of lung cancer in nonsmokers. A simple home test can tell you if the level of radon in your home is hazardous.

Your risk of developing lung cancer is higher if you're exposed to toxic substances such as asbestos or diesel exhaust in the workplace.

Other risk factors include:

- family history of lung cancer
- personal history of lung cancer, especially if you're a smoker
- previous radiation therapy to the chest

Home remedies for lung cancer symptoms

Home remedies and homeopathic remedies won't cure cancer. But certain home remedies may help relieve some of the symptoms associated with lung cancer and side effects of treatment.

Options may include:

Massage: With a qualified therapist, massage can help relieve pain and anxiety. Some massage therapists are trained to work with people with cancer.

Acupuncture: When performed by a trained practitioner, acupuncture may help ease pain, nausea, and vomiting. But it's not safe if you have low blood counts or take blood thinners.

Meditation: Relaxation and reflection can reduce stress and improve overall □uality of life in cancer patients.

Hypnosis: Helps you relax and may help with nausea, pain, and anxiety.

Yoga: Combining breathing techni□ues, meditation, and stretching, yoga can help you feel better overall and improve sleep.

Some people with cancer turn to cannabis oil. It can be infused into cooking oil to squirt in your mouth or mix with food. Or the vapors can be inhaled. This may relieve nausea and vomiting and improve appetite. Human studies are lacking and laws for use of cannabis oil vary from state to state.

Diet recommendations for people with lung cancer

There's no diet specifically for lung cancer. It is important to get all the nutrients your body needs. If you're deficient in certain vitamins or minerals, your doctor can advise you which foods can provide them. Otherwise, you'll need a dietary supplement. But don't take supplements without talking to your doctor because some can interfere with treatment.

Here are a few dietary tips:

- Eat whenever you have an appetite.
- If you don't have a major appetite, try eating smaller meals throughout the day.
- If you need to gain weight, supplement with low sugar, high-calorie foods and drinks.
- Use mint and ginger teas to soothe your digestive system.
- If your stomach is easily upset or you have mouth sores, avoid spices and stick to bland food.
- If constipation is a problem, add more high-fiber foods.

As you progress through treatment, your tolerance to certain foods may change. So can your side effects and nutritional needs. It's worth discussing nutrition with your doctor often. You can also ask for a referral to a nutritionist or dietician.

There's no diet known to cure cancer, but a well-balanced diet can help you fight side effects and feel better.

What specialists treat lung cancer?

The treatment of lung cancer requires a team approach. Surgical oncologists are surgeons specialized in the removal of cancers. Thoracic surgeons or general surgeons may also surgically treat lung cancers. Medical and radiation oncologists are specialists in the treatment of cancers with medications and radiation therapy, respectively. Other specialists who may be involved in the care of people with lung cancer include pain and palliative care specialists, as well as pulmonary specialists (medical pulmonologists).

How do health care professionals diagnose lung cancer?

Doctors use a wide range of diagnostic procedures and tests to diagnose lung cancer. These include the following:

The history and physical examination may reveal the presence of symptoms or signs that are suspicious for lung cancer. In addition to asking about symptoms and risk factors for cancer development such as smoking, doctors may detect signs of breathing difficulties, airway obstruction, or infections in the lungs. Cyanosis, a bluish color of the skin and the mucous membranes due to insufficient oxygen in the blood, suggests compromised function due to chronic disease of the lung. Likewise, changes in the tissue of the nail beds, known as clubbing, also may indicate chronic lung disease.

The chest X-ray is the most common first diagnostic step when any new symptoms of lung cancer are present. The chest X-ray procedure often involves a view from the back to the front of the chest as well as a view from the side. Like any X-ray procedure, chest X-rays expose the patient briefly to a small amount of radiation. Chest X-rays may reveal suspicious areas in the lungs but are unable to determine if these areas are cancerous. In particular, calcified nodules in the lungs or benign tumors called hamartomas may be identified on a chest X-ray and mimic lung cancer.

CT (computerized tomography) scans may be performed on the chest, abdomen, and/or brain to examine for both metastatic and lung tumors. CT scans are X-ray procedures that combine multiple images with the aid of a computer to generate cross-sectional views of the body. The images are taken by a large donut-shaped X-ray machine at different angles around the body. One advantage of CT scans is that they are more sensitive than standard chest X-rays in the detection of lung nodules, that is, they will demonstrate more nodules. Sometimes intravenous contrast material is given prior to the scan to help delineate the organs and their positions. The most common side effect is an adverse reaction to intravenous contrast material that may have been given prior to the procedure. This may result in itching, a rash, or hives that generally disappear rather □uickly. Severe anaphylactic reactions (life-threatening allergic reactions with breathing difficulties) to the contrast material are rare. CT scans of the abdomen may identify metastatic cancer in the liver or adrenal glands, and CT scans of the head may be ordered to reveal the presence and extent of metastatic cancer in the brain.

A technique called a low-dose helical CT scan (or spiral CT scan) is recommended by the USPSTF annually in current and former smokers between ages 55 and 80 with at least a 30 pack-year history of cigarette smoking who have smoked cigarettes within the past 15 years. The technique appears to increase the likelihood of detection of smaller, earlier, and more curable lung cancers. Three years of low-dose CT scanning in this group reduced the risk of lung cancer death by 20%. Use of models and rules for analyzing the results of these tests are decreasing the need for biopsy to evaluate detected nodules when the likelihood is high the nodule is not cancerous.

Magnetic resonance imaging (MRI) scans may be appropriate when precise detail about a tumor's location is required. The MRI technique uses magnetism, radio waves, and a computer to produce images of body structures. As with CT scanning, the patient is placed on a moveable bed which is inserted into the MRI scanner. There are no known side effects of MRI scanning, and there is no exposure to radiation. The image and resolution produced by MRI is □uite detailed and can detect tiny changes of structures within the body. People with heart pacemakers, metal implants, artificial heart valves, and other surgically implanted structures cannot be scanned with an MRI because of the risk that the magnet may move the metal parts of these structures.

Bone scans are used to create images of bones on a computer screen or on film. Doctors may order a bone scan to determine whether a lung cancer has metastasized to the bones. In a bone scan, a small amount of radioactive material is injected into the bloodstream and collects in the bones, especially in abnormal areas such as those involved by metastatic tumors. The radioactive material is detected by a scanner, and the image of the bones is recorded on a special film for permanent viewing.

Sputum cytology: The diagnosis of lung cancer always re□uires confirmation of malignant cells by a pathologist, even when symptoms and X-ray studies are suspicious for lung cancer. The simplest method to establish the diagnosis is the examination of sputum under a microscope. If a tumor is centrally located and has invaded the airways, this procedure, known as a sputum cytology examination, may allow visualization of tumor cells for diagnosis. This is the most risk-free and inexpensive tissue diagnostic procedure, but its value is limited since tumor cells will not always be present in sputum even if a cancer is present. Also, noncancerous cells may occasionally undergo changes in reaction to inflammation or injury that makes them look like cancer cells.

Bronchoscopy: Examination of the airways by bronchoscopy (visualizing the airways through a thin, fiberoptic probe inserted through the nose or mouth) may reveal areas of tumor that can be sampled (biopsied) for diagnosis by a pathologist. A tumor in the central areas of the lung or arising from the larger airways is accessible to sampling using this technique. Bronchoscopy may be performed using a rigid or a flexible fiberoptic bronchoscope and can be performed in a same-day outpatient bronchoscopy suite, an operating room, or on a hospital ward. The procedure can be uncomfortable, and it requires sedation or anesthesia. While bronchoscopy is relatively safe, it must be carried out by a lung specialist (pulmonologist or surgeon) experienced in the procedure. When a tumor is visualized and ade☐uately sampled, an accurate cancer diagnosis usually is possible. Some patients may cough up dark-brown blood for one to two days after the procedure. More serious but rare complications include a greater amount of bleeding, decreased levels of oxygen in the blood, and heart arrhythmias as well as complications from sedative medications and anesthesia.

Needle biopsy: Fine-needle aspiration (FNA) through the skin, most commonly performed with radiological imaging for guidance, may be useful in retrieving cells for diagnosis from tumor nodules in the lungs. Needle biopsies are particularly useful when the lung tumor is peripherally located in the lung and not accessible to sampling by bronchoscopy. A small amount of local anesthetic is given prior to insertion of a thin needle through the chest wall into the abnormal area in the lung. Cells are suctioned into the syringe and are examined under the microscope for tumor cells. This procedure is generally accurate when the tissue from the affected area is ade□uately sampled, but in some cases, adjacent or uninvolved areas of the lung may be mistakenly sampled. A small risk (3%-5%) of an air leak from the lungs (called a pneumothorax, which can easily be treated) accompanies the procedure.

Thoracentesis: Sometimes lung cancers involve the lining tissue of the lungs (pleura) and lead to an accumulation of fluid in the space between the lungs and chest wall (called a pleural effusion). Aspiration of a sample of this fluid with a thin needle (thoracentesis) may reveal the cancer cells and establish the diagnosis. As with the needle biopsy, a small risk of a pneumothorax is associated with this procedure.

Major surgical procedures: If none of the aforementioned methods yields a diagnosis, surgical methods must be employed to obtain tumor tissue for diagnosis. These can include mediastinoscopy (examining the chest cavity between the lungs through a surgically inserted probe with biopsy of tumor masses or lymph nodes that may contain metastases) or thoracotomy (surgical opening of the chest wall for removal or biopsy of a tumor). With a thoracotomy, it is rare to be able to completely remove a lung cancer, and both mediastinoscopy and thoracotomy carry the risks of major surgical procedures (complications such as bleeding, infection, and risks from anesthesia and medications). These procedures are performed in an operating room, and the patient must be hospitalized.

Blood tests: While routine blood tests alone cannot diagnose lung cancer, they may reveal biochemical or metabolic abnormalities in the body that accompany cancer. For example, elevated levels of calcium or of the enzyme alkaline phosphatase may accompany cancer that is metastatic to the bones. Likewise, elevated levels of certain enzymes normally present within liver cells, including aspartate aminotransferase (AST or SGOT) and alanine aminotransferase (ALT or SGPT), signal liver damage, possibly through the presence of tumor metastatic to the liver. One current focus of research in the area of lung cancer is the development of a blood test to aid in the diagnosis of lung cancer. Researchers have preliminary data that has identified specific proteins, or biomarkers, that are in the blood and may signal that lung cancer is present in someone with a suspicious area seen on a chest X-ray or other imaging study.

 Molecular testing: For advanced NSCLCs, molecular genetic testing is carried out to look for genetic mutations in the tumor. Mutations that are responsible for tumor growth are known as driver mutations. For example, testing may be done to look for mutations or abnormalities in the epithelial growth factor receptor (EGFR) and the anaplastic lymphoma kinase (ALK) genes. Other genes that may be mutated include MAPK and PIK3. Specific therapies are available that may be administered to patients whose tumors have these alterations in their genes.

Lung Cancer Symptoms, Stages, Treatment

How do health care professionals determine lung cancer staging?

The stage of a cancer is a measure of the extent to which a cancer has spread in the body. Staging involves evaluation of a cancer's size and its penetration into surrounding tissue as well as the presence or absence of metastases in the lymph nodes or other organs. Staging is important for determining how a particular cancer should be treated, since lung cancer therapies are geared toward specific stages. Staging of a cancer also is critical in estimating the prognosis of a given patient, with higher-stage cancers generally having a worse prognosis than lower-stage cancers.

Doctors may use several tests to accurately stage a lung cancer, including laboratory (blood chemistry) tests, X-rays, CT scans, bone scans, MRI scans, and PET scans. Abnormal blood chemistry tests may signal the presence of metastases in bone or liver, and radiological procedures can document the size of a cancer as well as its spread.

NSCLC are assigned a stage from I to IV in order of severity:

In stage I, the cancer is confined to the lung.

In stages II and III, the cancer is confined to the chest (with larger and more invasive tumors classified as stage III).

Stage IV cancer has spread from the chest to other parts of the body.

Most doctors use a two-tiered system to determine treatment for SCLC:

Limited-stage (LS) SCLC refers to cancer that is confined to its area of origin in the chest.

In extensive-stage (ES) SCLC, the cancer has spread beyond the chest to other parts of the body.

What is the treatment for lung cancer?

Treatment for lung cancer primarily involves surgical removal of the cancer, chemotherapy, or radiation therapy, as well as combinations of these treatments. Targeted therapies and immunotherapy are becoming more common, as well. The decision about which treatments will be appropriate for a given individual must take into account the location and extent of the tumor, as well as the overall health status of the patient.

As with other cancers, therapy may be prescribed that is intended to be curative (removal or eradication of a cancer) or palliative (measures that are unable to cure a cancer but can reduce pain and suffering). More than one type of therapy may be prescribed. In such cases, the therapy that is added to enhance the effects of the primary therapy is referred to as adjuvant therapy. An example of adjuvant therapy is chemotherapy or radiotherapy administered after surgical removal of a tumor in an attempt to kill any tumor cells that remain following surgery.

Surgery: Surgical removal of the tumor is generally performed for limited-stage (stage I or sometimes stage II) NSCLC and is the treatment of choice for cancer that has not spread beyond the lung. About 10%-35% of lung cancers can be removed surgically, but removal does not always result in a cure, since the tumors may already have spread and can recur at a later time. Among people who have an isolated, slow-growing lung cancer removed, 25%-40% are still alive five years after diagnosis. It is important to note that although a tumor may be anatomically suitable for resection, surgery may not be possible if the person has other serious conditions (such as severe heart or lung disease) that would limit their ability to survive an operation. Surgery is less often performed with SCLC than with NSCLC because these tumors are less likely to be localized to one area that can be removed.

The surgical procedure chosen depends upon the size and location of the tumor. Surgeons must open the chest wall and may perform a wedge resection of the lung (removal of a portion of one lobe), a lobectomy (removal of one lobe), or a pneumonectomy (removal of an entire lung). Sometimes lymph nodes in the region of the lungs also are removed (lymphadenectomy). Surgery for lung cancer is a major surgical procedure that re□uires general anesthesia, hospitalization, and follow-up care for weeks to months. Following the surgical procedure, patients may experience difficulty breathing, shortness of breath, pain, and weakness. The risks of surgery include complications due to bleeding, infection, and complications of general anesthesia.

Radiation: Radiation therapy may be employed as a treatment for both NSCLC and SCLC. Radiation therapy uses high-energy X-rays or other types of radiation to kill dividing cancer cells. Radiation therapy may be given as curative therapy, palliative therapy (using lower doses of radiation than with curative therapy), or as adjuvant therapy in combination with surgery or chemotherapy. The radiation is either delivered externally, by using a machine that directs radiation toward the cancer, or internally through placement of radioactive substances in sealed containers within the area of the body where the tumor is localized. Brachytherapy is a term used to describe the use of a small pellet of radioactive material placed directly into the cancer or into the airway next to the cancer. This is usually done through a bronchoscope.

Radiation therapy can be given if a person refuses surgery, if a tumor has spread to areas such as the lymph nodes or trachea making surgical removal impossible, or if a person has other conditions that make them too ill to undergo major surgery. Radiation therapy generally only shrinks a tumor or limits its growth when given as a sole therapy, yet in 10%-15% of people it leads to long-term remission and palliation of the cancer. Combining radiation therapy with chemotherapy can further prolong survival when chemotherapy is administered. A person who has severe lung disease in addition to a lung cancer may not be able to receive radiotherapy to the lung since the radiation can further decrease function of the lungs. A type of external radiation therapy called the "gamma knife" is sometimes used to treat single brain metastases. In this procedure, multiple beams of radiation coming from different directions are focused on the tumor over a few minutes to hours while the head is held in place by a rigid frame. This reduces the dose of radiation that is received by noncancerous tissues.

For external radiation therapy, a process called simulation is necessary prior to treatment. Using CT scans, computers, and precise measurements, simulation maps out the exact location where the radiation will be delivered, called the treatment field or port. This process usually takes 30 minutes to two hours. The external radiation treatment itself generally is done four or five days a week for several weeks.

SCLC often spreads to the brain. Sometimes people with SCLC that is responding well to treatment are treated with radiation therapy to the head to treat very early spread to the brain (called micrometastasis) that is not yet detectable with CT or MRI scans and has not yet produced symptoms. This is known as prophylactic brain radiation. Brain radiation therapy can cause short-term memory problems, fatigue, nausea, and other side effects.

Radiation therapy does not carry the risks of major surgery, but it can have unpleasant side effects, including fatigue and lack of energy. A reduced white blood cell count (rendering a person more susceptible to infection) and low blood platelet levels (making blood clotting more difficult and resulting in excessive bleeding) also can occur with radiation therapy. If the digestive organs are in the field exposed to radiation, patients may experience nausea, vomiting, or diarrhea. Radiation therapy can irritate the skin in the area that is treated, but this irritation generally improves with time after treatment has ended.

Chemotherapy: Both NSCLC and SCLC may be treated with chemotherapy. Chemotherapy refers to the administration of drugs that stop the growth of cancer cells by killing them or preventing them from dividing. Chemotherapy may be given alone, as an adjuvant to surgical therapy, or in combination with radiotherapy. While a number of chemotherapeutic drugs have been developed, the class of drugs known as the platinum-based drugs have been the most effective in treatment of lung cancers.

Chemotherapy is the treatment of choice for most SCLC, since these tumors are generally widespread in the body when they are diagnosed. Only half of people who have SCLC survive for four months without chemotherapy. With chemotherapy, their survival time is increased up to four- to fivefold. Chemotherapy alone is not particularly effective in treating NSCLC, but when NSCLC has metastasized, it can prolong survival in many cases.

Chemotherapy may be given as pills, as an intravenous infusion, or as a combination of the two. Chemotherapy treatments usually are given in an outpatient setting. A combination of drugs is given in a series of treatments, called cycles, over a period of weeks to months, with breaks in between cycles. Unfortunately, the drugs used in chemotherapy also kill normally dividing cells in the body, resulting in unpleasant side effects. Damage to blood cells can result in increased susceptibility to infections and difficulties with blood clotting (bleeding or bruising easily). Other side effects include fatigue, weight loss, hair loss, nausea, vomiting, diarrhea, and mouth sores. The side effects of chemotherapy vary according to the dosage and combination of drugs used and may also vary from individual to individual. Medications have been developed that can treat or prevent many of the side effects of chemotherapy. The side effects generally disappear during the recovery phase of the treatment or after its completion.

Targeted therapy: Molecularly targeted therapy involves the administration of drugs that have been identified to work in subsets of patients whose tumors have specific genetic changes (driver mutations) that promote tumor growth.

EGFR-targeted therapies: The drugs erlotinib (Tarceva), afatinib (Gilotrif), and gefitinib (Iressa) are so-called targeted drugs that more specifically target cancer cells, resulting in less damage to normal cells than general chemotherapeutic agents. Erlotinib, gefitinib, and afatinib target a protein called the epidermal growth factor receptor (EGFR) that is important in promoting the division of cells. The gene encoding this protein is mutated in many cases of non-small cell lung cancer, creating a mutation that encourages tumor growth. Mutations in the EGFR gene are more common in cancers in women and in people who have never smoked. Drugs that target the EGFR receptor sometimes stop working after a time, which is known as resistance to the drug. Resistance often occurs because the cancer has developed a new mutation in the same gene, and a common example of this is the so-called EGFR T790M mutation. Some newer EGFR-targeted drugs also work against cells with the T790M mutation, including osimertinib (Tagrisso). Necitumumab (Portrazza) is another drug that targets EGFR. It can be used along with chemotherapy as the first treatment in people with advanced NSCLC of the s☐uamous cell type.

Other targeted therapies: Other targeted drugs are available that target other driver mutations. These other targeted therapies include the ALK tyrosine kinase inhibitor drugs crizotinib (Xalkori), alectinib (Alecensa), brigatinib (Alunbrig), and ceritinib (Zykadia) that are used in patients whose tumors have an abnormality of the ALK gene as the driver mutation. Some of these drugs may also be helpful for people whose cancers have an abnormality of the gene known as ROS1.

The gene known as BRAF can also be abnormal in lung cancers causing the production of BRAF protein that promotes the cancer's growth. Dabrafenib (Tafinlar) is a type of drug known as a BRAF inhibitor and attacks the BRAF protein directly. Trametinib (Mekinist) is known as a MEK inhibitor because it attacks MEK proteins, which are related to BRAF proteins. These may be used for patients with tumors that have abnormal BRAF genes.

Other attempts at targeted therapy include drugs known as antiangiogenesis drugs, which block the development of new blood vessels within a cancer. Without adequate blood vessels to supply oxygen-carrying blood, the cancer cells will die. The antiangiogenic drug bevacizumab (Avastin) has also been found to prolong survival in advanced lung cancer when it is added to the standard chemotherapy regimen. Bevacizumab is given intravenously every two to three weeks. However, since this drug may cause bleeding, it is not appropriate for use in patients who are coughing up blood, if the lung cancer has spread to the brain, or in people who are receiving anticoagulation therapy ("blood thinner" medications). Bevacizumab also is not used in cases of s☐uamous cell cancer because it leads to bleeding from this type of lung cancer. Ramucirumab (Cyramza) is another angiogenesis inhibitor that can be used to treat advanced non-small cell lung cancer.

Immunotherapy: Immunotherapy may be an effective option for some patients with advanced lung cancers. Immunotherapy drugs work by strengthening the activity of the immune system against tumor cells. The immunotherapy drugs nivolumab (Opdivo) and pembrolizumab (Keytruda) were approved by the U.S. FDA in 2015 for the treatment of lung cancer. These drugs are checkpoint inhibitors that target checkpoints or areas that control the immune response and promote the immune response. These two drugs target the PD-1 protein, which strengthens the immune response against the cancers. Atezolizumab (Tecentriq) is a drug that targets PD-L1, a protein related to PD-1 that is found on some tumor cells and immune cells.

Radiofre☐uency ablation (RFA): Radiofre☐uency ablation is being studied as an alternative to surgery, particularly in cases of early stage lung cancer. In this type of treatment, a needle is inserted through the skin into the cancer, usually under guidance by CT scanning. Radiofrequency (electrical) energy is then transmitted to the tip of the needle where it produces heat in the tissues, killing the cancerous tissue and closing small blood vessels that supply the cancer. RFA usually is not painful and has been approved by the FDA for the treatment of certain cancers, including lung cancers. Studies have shown that this treatment can prolong survival similarly to surgery when used to treat early stages of lung cancer but without the risks of major surgery and the prolonged recovery time associated with major surgical procedures.

Experimental therapies: Since no therapy is currently available that is absolutely effective in treating lung cancer, patients may be offered a number of new therapies that are still in the experimental stage, meaning that doctors do not yet have enough information to decide whether these therapies should become accepted forms of treatment for lung cancer. New drugs or new combinations of drugs are tested in so-called clinical trials, which are studies that evaluate the effectiveness of new medications in comparison with those treatments already in widespread use. Newer types of immunotherapy are being studied that involve the use of vaccine-related therapies that attempt to utilize the body's immune system to directly fight cancer cells. Lung cancer treatment vaccines are being studied in clinical trials.

What is the prognosis and life expectancy of lung cancer?

The prognosis of lung cancer refers to the chance for cure or prolongation of life (survival) and is dependent upon where the cancer is located, the size of the cancer, the presence of symptoms, the type of lung cancer, and the overall health status of the patient.

SCLC has the most aggressive growth of all lung cancers, with a median survival time of only two to four months after diagnosis when untreated. (That is, by two to four months, half of all patients have died.) However, SCLC is also the type of lung cancer most responsive to radiation therapy and chemotherapy. Because SCLC spreads rapidly and is usually disseminated at the time of diagnosis, methods such as surgical removal or localized radiation therapy are less effective in treating this type of lung cancer. When chemotherapy is used alone or in combination with other methods, survival time can be prolonged four- to fivefold; however, of all patients with SCLC, only 5%-10% are still alive five years after diagnosis. Most of those who survive have limited-stage SCLC before treatment.

In non-small cell lung cancer (NSCLC), the most important prognostic factor is the stage (extent of spread) of the tumor at the time of diagnosis. Results of standard treatment are generally poor in all but the smallest of cancers that can be surgically removed. However, in stage I cancers that can be completely removed surgically, five-year survival approaches 75%. Radiation therapy can produce a cure in a small minority of patients with NSCLC and leads to relief of symptoms in most patients. In advanced-stage disease, chemotherapy offers modest improvements in survival although rates of overall survival are poor.

The overall prognosis for lung cancer is poor when compared with some other cancers. Survival rates for lung cancer are generally lower than those for most cancers, with an overall five-year survival rate for lung cancer of about 17% compared to 65% for colon cancer, 91% for breast cancer, 81% for bladder cancer, and over 99% for prostate cancer.

Is it possible to prevent lung cancer?

Cessation of smoking and eliminating exposure to tobacco smoke is the most important measure that can prevent lung cancer. Many products, such as nicotine gum, nicotine sprays, or nicotine inhalers, may be helpful to people trying to □uit smoking. Minimizing exposure to passive smoking also is an effective preventive measure. Using a home radon test kit can identify and allow correction of increased radon levels in the home. Methods that allow early detection of cancers, such as the helical low-dose CT scan, also may be of value in the identification of small cancers that can be cured by surgical resection and prevented from becoming widespread, incurable, metastatic cancer.

WHAT IS CBD OIL

Suddenly, cannabidiol (CBD) oil seems to be everywhere. People are dropping it into their nighttime tea, swallowing capsules, and loading it into their vape pens, claiming it relieves depression, masks chronic pain, and helps them sleep deeper. And although CBD oil is often derived from marijuana plants, it won't get you high and it's not just pot users who are partaking.

But what is CBD oil, exactly? CBD oil is typically extracted from the resin glands on cannabis (marijuana) buds and flowers. It can also be extracted from hemp, which is an industrial, fibrous form of cannabis that has small buds and a tetrahydrocannabinol, or THC, concentration of 0.3% or less (THC is the chemical compound that's responsible for making people high). It's usually diluted with another type of oil, like MCT oil."Cannabidiol (CBD) is one of over 80 phytocannabinoids, or chemical compounds, produced by the cannabis plant," says Sarah Cohen, secretary, R.N., of the American Cannabis Nurses Association. CBD oil is what you get when you take cannabinoids from cannabis and mix them with a carrier oil, like MCT (a form of coconut oil), explains Devin O'Dea, the chief marketing officer at MINERAL Health. Until recently, THC (or tetrahydrocannabinol), the compound in cannabis that gets you high, was the most well-known element of the plant—but now CBD is giving THC a run for its money. CBD is legal in all the states where medical marijuana is legal (30 states plus the District of Columbia have laws allowing it to some extent, mostly for medicinal purposes), as well as an additional 16 states.

Is CBD marijuana?

CBD oil is a cannabinoid derived from the cannabis plant. Until recently, the most well-known compound in cannabis was delta-9 tetrahydrocannabinol (THC). This is the most active ingredient in marijuana. Marijuana contains both THC and CBD, but the compounds have different effects. THC is well-known for the mind-altering "high" it produces when broken down by heat and introduced into the body, such as when smoking the plant or cooking itinto foods. Unlike THC, CBD is not psychoactive. This means that it does not change the state of mind of the person who uses it. However, it does appear to produce significant changes in the body and has been found to have medical benefits. Most of the CBD used medicinally is found in the least processed form of the cannabis plant, known as hemp. Hemp and marijuana come from the same plant, cannabis sativa, but they are very different. Over the years, marijuana farmers have selectively bred their plants to be very high in THC and other compounds that interested them, either for a smell or an effect they had on the plant's flowers. On the other hand, hemp farmers have not tended to modify the plant. It is these hemp plants that are used to create CBD oil.

The Guide to Cannabinoids in Cannabis

The field of cannabis research is vast and diverse. From biochemical studies of the plant itself to physiological and chemical studies of its pharmacology to psychological and social research into its effects, researchers' studying cannabis produce the knowledge at the foundation of industry innovation and public policy. Yet perhaps the most important research being done in this new era of expanded access to legal cannabis pertains to just one facet of the plant: the humble cannabinoid. Cannabinoids, the chemicals that □ualify the plant as a drug, are the sine □ua non of the commercial and medical significance of cannabis. Despite their importance, however, our scientific understanding of cannabinoids has been stunted, in the United States, by prohibition and elsewhere, by restrictive regulations. The result is a literature on the subject that's patchy and inconsistent, yet reflective of the market's interest in THC and CBD. Toppling regulations and expanding legalization, however, have made it possible for researchers to conduct more thorough investigations into other cannabinoids. Exploring the world of cannabinoids can be rewarding for anyone interested in cultivating a more intentional relationship with cannabis. Knowledge about precisely how and why certain strains and products produce their effects is empowering. For those ready to take the plunge, here's the ultimate guide to the cannabinoids in cannabis. We start with an overview of cannabinoids in general, how and why they react with our bodies, and then dive into the most important cannabinoids. As a bonus for all you vape-fans and dab-heads, we list the boiling point for each cannabinoid for easy reference.

What is a Cannabinoid?

Cannabinoids get their name less from what they are and more from what they do. They're a class of chemical compounds the cannabis plant naturally produces. But they have the uni☐ue property of being able to interact with receptors in our cells. These interactions, through a complex series of pathways, alter the release of chemicals in the brain. These alterations, in turn, produce a wide array of effects throughout the body. According to a recent tally, scientists have successfully isolated 113 discrete cannabinoids. Many of them exhibit their own distinct effects. Of those 113, THC, CBD and CBN have the most substantial body of research behind them. CBD and CBN were to first cannabinoids researchers identified when they discovered cannabinoids in the 1940s. It would take until 1964 for researchers to correctly determine the structure of THC. From a scientific and legal perspective, there's a difference between the cannabinoids the plant naturally produces and those produced synthetically. The former are called "phytocannabinoids."

Is Cannabis Therapy Worth the Risk?

Because scientists are driven by data, few doctors or researchers are willing to recommend cannabis to treat autism. In contrast to epilepsy, which has references dating back as far as 1843, there just isn't a sufficient body of evidence for most physicians to feel comfortable recommending cannabis as a treatment. Piomelli cautions that dosing can be problematic, that many parents may not be e□uipped to assess or monitor proper dosing, and that attempting to do so without the guidance of a □ualified professional could have serious consequences: "[P]harmacology is all about doses. Low doses can be good, while high doses can be bad. One thing people need to understand is that if the endocannabinoid system has a protective role, it doesn't mean that activating this system may not be harmful."

He cautions there is a possibility one risks "messing up the endocannabinoid system. Even though the intent is to enhance social behavior, one may end up actually having the opposite effect. "Further, because we're dealing with plants, there are added layers of complexity. Whereas, with most pharmacological drugs, there is usually a single active compound to treat a condition, cannabis contains potentially hundreds. This can be a good thing or a bad thing. Many attribute the efficacy of cannabis to an entourage effect—or a synergy between ingredients. While this may be an overall positive, it doesn't lessen the complexity of determining which component may be helping, and which may be counterproductive or harmful."

HOW CAN CANNABIS OIL HELP YOU?

Cannabis oil can help you if you are a cancer patient who does not take "we have done all we can do" to heart, but instead looks for an alternate method. Or maybe you aren't convinced that Western medicine practices are right for you. With safe, high □uality cannabis oil, you are providing yourself with improvements in your well-being and your standard of living in regards to pain management. As mentioned above, there are numerous diseases and conditions that can be treated using cannabis oil. It is ultimately up to the patient to make the decision what route he or she wants to make: Western practices, alternative methods or a combination of both, like the Cancer patient did by undergoing surgery and then deciding the cannabis oil route was for her. And look at where she ended up.

Not only did she digest the cannabis oil, but she topically applied it to the two spots of skin cancer on her collar bone. She started to see notable differences on her skin within 48 hours, and in the patient's case the spots appeared to be gone in over a week. She continued to ingest the cannabis oil and two weeks later, the pain she been experiencing for years was almost non-existent. She continued to ingest cannabis oil on a daily basis and slowly started to increase the amount she was taking.

Just over one year later from her initial diagnosis, the patient returned to her doctor to see if the effects of the cannabis oil had been working like she had hoped it would. He examined her, not once, not twice, but three times before he told her the news. He said, "It's gone! I can't find anything at all. If it wasn't for the scar tissue I would never have known you had ever had cancer." Needless to say patient was in disbelief that cannabis oil had been the one to lead her back to her normal, everyday lifestyle.

Cannabis Entourage Effect: Why Whole Plant Medicine Matters

Piomelli, like most doctors, would not recommend cannabis as a treatment, because there is little scientific research to base it on. Unlike epilepsy, the research on autism is in its infancy. However, recognizing that parents who've tried everything see cannabis as a last defense, "I certainly would not pass judgment on a parent who is desperate and would do it. I'm just saying be very, very careful what you do." Other professionals privately admit that for parents who feel they've exhausted all other options, the unknowns and potential risks may be acceptable. According to the late Bernard Rimland, founder of the Autism Society of America and former director of the Autism Research Institute, "the benefit/risk profile of medical marijuana seems fairly benign" when compared to Risperdal or what Dr. Rimland considers the least useful and most dangerous: psychotropic drugs.

"Moreover, the reports we are seeing from parents indicate that medical marijuana often works when no other treatments, drug or non-drug, have helped," Rimland added.

CBD oil Dosage Lung cancer

Especially relevant is that the dosage amount should be mostly determined by the severity of the condition. Secondly, you should take the size (age) of your kid into consideration. Cannabidiol is also safe to experiment with different dosages.

 According to CBD experts, and scientific reports, it is not possible to overdose with CBD. However, The Pediatric Cannabis Support recommends for starters to go with the low usage dose and increase it gradually. Oral intake is the most common way of CBD consumption for autism. Besides that, when kids are sensitive to certain tastes, mixing it with food is a very popular way of consumption. Sometimes sprays are also used.

 From parent reports of autistic children of 10 years and older treated with CBD, we hear that a CBD autism dosing of 25 mg taken twice a day is a good way to start. From parent reports of small autistic children (younger than 5 years) treated with CBD, we hear that a CBD autism dosing of 10 mg taken twice a day is a good way to start. When parents are monitoring for four days before changing dosage levels (like increasing when symptoms only mildly reduced), they can determine what dosage level works best for their child. Take into account that some symptoms (like mood and focus) improve more or less instantly, other symptoms like being non-verbal can take weeks to slowly erode. Speach does not return (or start) immediately.

In cancer treatment, CBD oil is supporting weed oil, when mixed together. Dosing is also, in this case, crucial and we have highlighted several dosage roadmaps in our Delta-9-THC oil dosage. One of the most common uses of CBD oil is to mitigate pain and anxiety. Therefore we have tested some oils to find the best CBD oil for pain and the best CBD oil for anxiety. If you are lost when it comes to determining how many drops of CBD oil for any given milligram dosing amount, you might find our CBD Dosage Calculator helpful.

Everyday Advanced CBD Dose Titration for Children

For pediatric dose titration, start with one drop, 3 times per day. If well tolerated go to 2 drops, wait a few days. If no adverse effects are noted, you can go the therapeutic starting dose with is 4 drops 3X per day.

A good starting point for general pediatric CBD dosing is to start with .5mg CBD per pound of body weight, split across 3 doses per day. This is a therapeutic dose that you can increase under medical supervision and in response to the therapeutic need. CBD has a stellar safety profile but all cannabis products are biphasic which means they could have significant side effects at both very low or very high doses. Use of CBD to treat pediatric epilepsy could employ a 5-10X higher dose but this is obviously an extreme use case. Each condition I treat with CBD necessitates an individual prescription for the patient to achieve exact dose titration. Example: A 70-pound child should take 35-40 mg of CBD per day, split over 3 doses taken with food. 4 drops of Everyday Advanced will yield 12.5 mg of CBD.

Everyday Advanced CBD Dose Titration for Adults

A starting dose of CBD for a 140-pound adult is 1.2 to 1.8 ml of oil per day to yield a daily dose of 60-90 mg of CBD. The Everyday Advanced label suggest taking .6ml (one-eighth of a teaspoon) two to three times a day, which provides 30 mg of CBD per dose. Example: A 140-pound adult should take 70 mg of CBD daily (.5mg of CBD per pound of body weight) split over 3 doses taken with food. If desired results are not obtained and the CBD is well tolerated, you can double the dose after one-week and then wait two weeks. If you again have not achieved the desired results you can go as high as 2mg/pound/day.

www.ingramcontent.com/pod-product-compliance
Lightning Source LLC
Chambersburg PA
CBHW061729250726
48657CB00002B/837